Vitex

The Women's Herb

Christopher Hobbs, L.Ac.

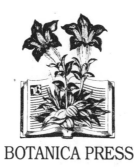

BOTANICA PRESS

This book is printed on recycled paper

Look for these books by Christopher Hobbs—
available from Botanica Press:

The Herbs and Health Series:

Echinacea! The Immune Herb
Foundations of Health
Ginkgo, Elixir of Youth
Handbook for Herbal Healing
Kombucha, Manchurian Tea Mushroom
Medicinal Mushrooms
Milk Thistle, The Liver Herb
Natural Liver Therapy
The Ginsengs, A User's Guide
Usnea, Herbal Antibiotic
Valerian, The Relaxing and Sleep Herb

NEW!
Christopher Hobbs' Herbal Prescriber (herbs on disk)

6th Printing - July, 1996
Second Edition

Copyright October, 1990

Michael Miovic, editor
Beth Baugh, copy editor
Michael Amster, research assistant
Illustrations: fig. 1 Cazin, fig. 2 Mark Johnson

Photographs: fig. 3-5 Christopher Hobbs

Special thanks to Madaus Co. for
supplying German translations

BOTANICA PRESS, 10226 Empire Grade, Santa Cruz, CA 95060

Table of Contents

$\mathcal{I}$NTRODUCTION

$\mathcal{T}$he use of herbs to heal our health problems, ease pains, and increase vigor and well-being goes back to the dawn of history. Today herbal medicine is still one of the most important methods of healing in many cultures throughout the world—and it is now gaining new acceptance in our own modern, scientific culture. In the last fifty to one-hundred years, an increasing number of herbal medicines have been studied in clinics and laboratories and found to be effective. One such plant is vitex, which is prized for its ability to restore balance to the female hormonal system. Throughout Europe, where herbal medicine has more of an unbroken tradition than it does in the United States, vitex is the number one herb to help relieve the symptoms of female hormonal imbalances such as the depression, cramps, mood swings, water retention, weight gain, and other PMS symptoms associated with the menstrual cycle. Vitex extracts are also prescribed for uterine fibroid cysts and to help ease the symptoms of menopause.

This booklet will explain everything you might want to know about vitex—both its traditional and modern uses, as well as what the latest scientific findings are on this

remarkable herb. You'll also find lots of practical and easy-to-understand information which you can put to use right away—things like:
- Which ailments vitex is good for
- How vitex works
- Choosing the best vitex product
- How much vitex to take and for how long

In this revised edition, there is a special appendix that summarizes scientific details about the botany, chemistry, pharmacology, toxicology, pharmacy, and cultivation of vitex. In addition, the appendix examines the debate surrounding the safety and efficacy of synthetic hormone replacement therapy. A thorough reference list is attached for further reading on women's health.

THE HISTORY OF VITEX

Vitex is native to Greece and Italy and was well-known by the ancients. The name "vitex" comes from the Romans, perhaps because the plant's leaves and its flexible branches looked like willow, *salix*, and like willow were used in wickerwork (Jones, 1956).

The scientific name for vitex, *Vitex agnus-castus*, comes from the Greek *agnos castus*, meaning "chaste," because the ancient Greeks thought the plant calmed the sexual passions. Pliny, the great Greek natural historian (AD 23-79), wrote that the plant "checks violent sexual desire" and that it was valued highly for many different health problems. For instance, a drink made from the seeds of vitex was taken to reduce fevers and headaches and to stimulate perspiration, as well as to

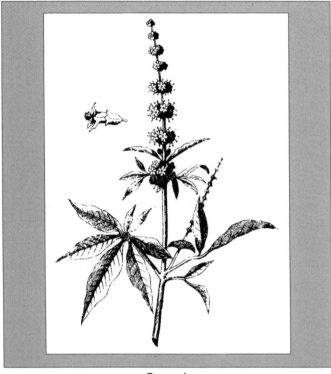

Figure I

promote menstruation, "to purge the uterus," and to promote the flow of milk in new mothers. Because of their hot nature, vitex seeds were taken to dispel "wind" or flatulence from the bowels, promote urination, check diarrhea, and ameliorate dropsy and splenic diseases. Both the seeds and the leaves were also considered efficacious against the bites of spiders and snakes, and for the latter remedy, two tender leaves of vitex were taken in wine or in a mixture of vinegar and water.

After the fall of Rome, Western medicine went into hibernation for awhile. Throughout the Middle Ages medical writers in Europe simply recopied the ancient Greek and Roman sources. However, original medical thought did flourish in Persia during the "Golden Age" of

Arabic science, and this heritage has been preserved in
the works of several notable authors. Two important
works of the time are available in English editions, *The
Medical Formulary of Al-Samarquandi* (Levy and Al-
Khaledy, 1967), from about 1200 AD, and *The Medical
Formulary of Al-Kindi* (Levy, 1967). These works show
that *agnus castus* was known to the Persians. Both
authors say vitex was used with other herbs to cure
insanity, madness, and epilepsy. In fact, the fruits of
vitex are still sold today in Egyptian bazaars as *"a calm-
ing agent in hysteria"* (Levy, 1967).

The Renaissance in Europe brought a new wave of
interest in the medicinal arts. From the mid 1500s to the
mid 1600s, many important writers published works on
herbalism: in Germany, Boch, Fuchs, and Brunfels; in
England, Turner, Dodoens, Gerard, and Parkinson; and
in Italy, Matthioli. These books have come to be known
as "the great herbals."

Gerard, one of the greatest of the Renaissance herbalists, gathered information about the uses of herbs from
Greek and Roman sources, as well as from folk uses and
professional herbalists of the time (Gerard and Johnson,
1633). His information tends to be both fanciful and
practical. For example, on the fanciful side, he thought
that vitex would have the same effect whether taken as a
powder, tea, or worn on the body. Also, like many before
him, Gerard said that vitex is *the* remedy for those who
want to maintain chastity. On a more practical note,
however, he extolled vitex as a cure for flatulence and
recommended an infusion of the fruits in wine to *"cureth
the stoppings of the liver and spleen."* Significantly,
Gerard also encouraged its use as a "female" herb, writ-
ing that the seeds and leaves are good against pain and

inflammations of the uterus, while the seed drunk with pennyroyal will bring on the menses.

After the early 1700s, vitex fell out of popularity in England, where it wasn't rediscovered until it garnered new interest as an herb for female reproductive imbalances in the mid 1900s. The English author Grieve, in her famous *A Modern Herbal* (1931), gives vitex a scant paragraph or two, saying only that a tincture of the fresh, ripe berries can be used *"for the relief of paralysis, pains in the limbs, weakness, etc."*

However, in countries closer to the Mediterranean, where vitex grows naturally, the herb never lost its popularity entirely and was considered an effective remedy for many ailments, including colic, gas, and other digestive problems. For instance, in France, even through the 1880s, vitex fruits were used to promote good digestion and to remove "visceral obstructions." Cazin, the author of a French herbal treatise from the late 1800s, mentions that the use of vitex to cool the passions was well known, and he also mentions a syrup made from the seeds of vitex which was famous at the time as *"an infallible remedy for maintaining chastity and repressing the ardors of Venus."* Cazin goes on to say that this syrup was widely distributed in convents to subdue passion, but that he doubted it worked. In fact, he even thought that the vitex syrup had "a very stimulating property."

The modern interest in vitex began in Germany where, in 1930, Dr. Gerhard Madaus conducted some of the first scientific research on the plant's effect on the female hormonal system. Since then scientific interest in vitex has grown immensely and in 1986 was introduced into American herbal medicine. Table 1 summarizes the history of vitex.

TABLE 1: HISTORY OF VITEX AT A GLANCE

c. 450 B.C.	Hippocrates recommends vitex for injuries, inflammations, and enlargement of the spleen (Madaus, 1938).
c. 50 A.D.	Dioscorides says vitex is good for inflammations of the uterus.
c. 1200	From the medicine of the Persian school, Al-Kindi prescribes vitex for epilepsy.
c. 1530-1640	Gerard and other Renaissance herbalists recommend vitex for inflammation of the uterus and as an emmenagogue.
c. 1890	Cazin mentions the use of vitex for calming sexual passions.
1930	Madaus reports some of the first scientific findings on vitex.
1953	First clinical work on vitex's galactagogue activity.

MODERN PROVINGS

Because of the long and interesting history of vitex's use for female imbalances, in the 1930s, Dr. Gerhard Madaus developed a patent medicine from an extract of the dried vitex fruits. Madaus named this medicine *Agnolyt*[tm] and used it to begin scientific investigations of vitex. Since then most of the clinical and laboratory studies on vitex have been done with this preparation.

Using Agnolyt in the early 1950s, several researchers confirmed the age-old belief that vitex stimulates milk production (Hahn et al, 1984). In one carefully controlled study with one-hundred nursing mothers, it was found that women who took vitex had an increased milk flow and ease of milk-release as compared to women who took a placebo. Later research showed that the best way to stimulate milk production in new mothers is to have them start taking vitex the first day after birth and to continue taking it for at least ten days.

In the late 1950s, researchers were able to demonstrate that vitex specifically helps resolve menstrual disorders. In a study of 51 women who had heavy bleeding during menstruation and excessively short menstrual cycles, 65% of all of those who took Agnolyt^tm showed improvement. About 47% of the women were entirely cured (those over 20 seemed to have the highest cure rate), while 18% had at least some positive results. However, note that 35% of the women were not influenced by the vitex treatment—we will explain this finding in the section on Constitutional Types (Kayser and Istanbulluoglu, 1954).

Further clinical studies performed in the 1960s through early 1990s have clarified and completed the clinical picture about vitex. Table 2 summarizes the most important findings of this research. Note the table is a general review of research, therefore, a 'successful' finding or conclusion on a particular vitex study does not mean that all patients (100%) were cured of illness.

TABLE 2: SUMMARY OF CLINICAL FINDINGS ON VITEX (AGNOLYT)

ILLNESS OR IMBALANCE	*RESULTS & PROCEDURE*	*REFERENCES*
Various menstrual bleeding disorders (amenorrhea, hypermenorrhea, oligomenorrhea).	Strong rate of success. Patients usually require minimum of 3 months vitex therapy for effect.	Amman, 1982; Loch, 1990; Attelmann, 1972
Menstrual cycle irregularities due to previous progesterone therapy.	Successful treatment, reestablished regular cycle.	Attelmann, 1972; Brantner, 1979
Symptoms of PMS caused by hypersecretion of estrogen (emotional depression, migraine headaches, skin and other allergies, breast tenderness, cramps, colic, edema in lower calves, feeling of bloating).	Vitex provides relief of symptoms when taken for at least 6 months. For optimum effect, treatment should continue for an additional 3 to 6 months to avoid relapse.	Albus, 1966; Amman, 1965; Dittmar, 1989; Feldmann, 1996
Fibrocystic Disease	Positive results with a reduction of symptoms. Vitex taken for at least 3 months.	Grogle, 1979; Kubista, 1986
Premenopausal symptoms caused by reduced progesterone production.	Vitex stimulated the secretion of luteotropic hormone, thus increasing the output of progesterone.	Amman, 1974
Hyperprolactinemia	Overall success with vitex therapy.	Amberg, 1991; Milewica, 1993
Corpus Luteum insufficiency (CLI)	Vitex successfully treats the condition, reestablishing normal function of the ovaries.	Proppings, 1987; Fedlmann, 1995
Insufficient mild flow in nursing mothers	Vitex increased rates and ease of milk delivery for nursing mothers.	Hahn et al, 1984
Hormone-related jaw problems during puberty and nursing	Successful treatment with vitex.	Riemensperger, 1961

(*Table 2, continued on page 9*)

TABLE 2, CONTINUED FROM PAGE 8

ILLNESS OR IMBALANCE	RESULTS & PROCEDURE	REFERENCES
Acne during puberty (also in men)	Good results with vitex.	Amman, 1987; Giss, 1988
Hormonally-related constipation (caused by hyperestrogen in PMS)	Successful relief from long-standing constipation.	Amman, 1986

TABLE 3: MAJOR SYMPTOMS OF PMS

- Emotional depression
- Migraine headache
- Skin rashes, allergies, and acne
- Mastitis with special sensitivity of the breasts
- Uterine cramps
- False angina pectoris (heart pains)
- Abdominal cramping (dysmenorrhea)
- Edema of the lower legs with a sensation of puffiness
- Change in appetite

CONDITIONS
VITEX CAN TREAT

HOW VITEX WORKS

Modern clinical experience and research shows that
vitex can be extremely helpful in balancing the female
sexual hormones. Specifically, it can not only ease but,
with time, actually cure premenstrual syndrome (PMS),
which has been linked to abnormally high levels of
estrogen. Table 3 shows the major symptoms of PMS.
Vitex can be very helpful in relieving these symptoms,
especially if they disappear when menstruation begins
(Amann, 1975). Taken over a long period of time, vitex
can also help with other menstrual symptoms such as
heavy bleeding or too short a menstrual cycle. Table 4
lists some other important hormone-related imbalances
and conditions that vitex may successfully treat.

But how does vitex actually do all this?—Scientists
think that it works by regulating the pituitary gland,
which has been called the "master gland" because it is
the major control gland. The pituitary gland, well-pro-

tected deep under the front part of the brain, sends chemical signals to other glands such as the ovaries and "tells" them how much of a particular hormone to make. For instance, when there is too much estrogen in the blood, the pituitary detects these increased levels from sensors elsewhere in the body and tells the ovaries to make less of it, with the result that the amount of estrogen in the blood drops to normal levels. This effect is called *negative feedback*.

TABLE 4. OTHER CONDITIONS VITEX CAN TREAT

Any hormone-related symptoms in women that disappear with the onset of pregnancy and reappear after breastfeeding ends.

Amenorrhea (menstruation stops). See the section on Vitex and Pregnancy.

Irregular menstruation, especially if this condition is accompanied by endometriosis, or abnormal overgrowth of the uterus lining.

Uterine cysts (fibroid cysts) that occur in the smooth muscle tissue, or subserous layers of the uterine muscle. However, if the cyst occurs in a submucous area, vitex is less likely to be helpful.

After withdrawal from progesterone-containing pills, "the pill," taking vitex for several months may help stabilize the menstrual cycle and bring on ovulation more quickly.

To help stimulate milk-production in new mothers. See the section on "Vitex and Pregnancy".

Acne in teenagers, including young men. See the section on "Vitex and Acne".

Swelling of the knee during menstruation

Affection of the jaw joint, which may occur during puberty, lactation period, and menopause.

Treatment of painful sores on the tongue and mucous membranes of the mouth caused by *Herpes simplex recidivans* and *Stomatitis aphthosa ulcerosa* (Koch, undated).

Constipation due to PMS and excessive estrogen secretion (Amman, 1965).

Headache due to corpus luteum insufficieny and PMS (Ecker, 1964).

Vitex and Endometriosis

German gynecologists have reported remarkable success treating endometriosis with vitex. It is best used in the treatment of mild endometriosis, where vitex can help prevent advancement of the disease (Agnolyt Manual, 1994). In the treatment of advanced endometriosis with glandular-cystic hyperplasia, however, synthetic hormone progestational agents are required. The administration of hormones initiates menstruation, cleansing the diseased endometrious surface. Following this restoring of menstruation, the patient should begin vitex treatment to help prevent further complications.

Vitex and Pregnancy

Vitex can safely be taken throughout the end of the third month of pregnancy and may help prevent miscarriage, according to German research. After the third month it is still safe to take but is not recommended, because it may bring on the flow of milk too early.

I have also found that a formula of vitex, ginger, lavender, wild yam, and a little Chinese rhubarb may be helpful for morning sickness.

For women who are *trying* to get pregnant, vitex may be useful to help regulate the ovulatory cycle, if this or other sexual hormone imbalance is preventing pregnancy.

Vitex and Menopause

Because progesterone production decreases at the time of menopause, vitex may help reduce some of the undesirable symptoms that can occur at this time, such as vaginal dryness, hot flashes, dizziness, and depression. In fact, vitex and preparations containing the herb are the most widely-used natural medicine in Europe for

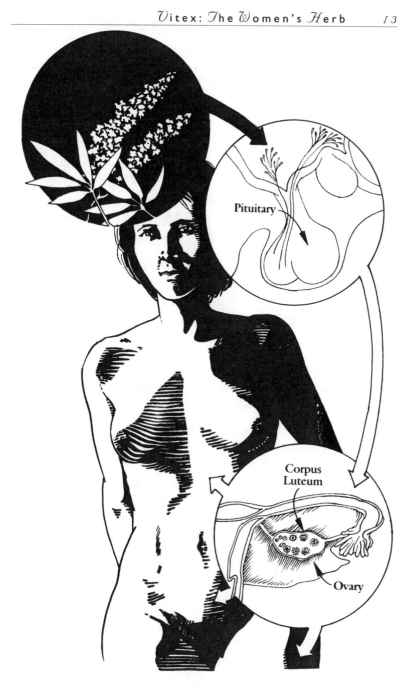

Figure 2

helping to relieve unpleasant symptoms that may occur before, during, and after menopause, being recommended by herbalists and physicians alike.

For these purposes, try combining vitex with other female tonic herbs such as saw palmetto fruits for supporting the nutrition of the female organs, dang gui for building the blood and female organs, black cohosh for regulating estrogen balance and helping to relieve hot flashes, and blue cohosh for relieving pelvic pain and congestion. David Hoffmann, a British-trained medical herbalist who has used vitex clinically for years, has reported that the most common use of vitex preparations in his experience throughout England, Wales, and Scotland is for symptoms of menopause (Personal communication, 1990).

Vitex and Acne

Several studies indicate that vitex can help control acne in teenagers, both among young women and men. As a clinician, I have been recommending vitex liquid drops to my acne patients for a number of years—with excellent results. I have sometimes found teenagers with acne to be especially difficult to work with, not because they are unfriendly or uncooperative, but because they often do not see the value of positive dietary changes. I have worked with some teenagers who had chronic acne for several years who were not willing to change their diet in any way. They felt attached to soft drinks, french fries, pizza and hamburgers, and no amount of logical discussion could change their minds. If vitex can help in these cases, it seems likely to help in other cases where dietary improvements are possible, and in my experience, it *can* help dramatically. I have given it to both young men and women with equal effectiveness. The remedy often takes from one to two months before it becomes fully active. I often add an herbal formula for "cooling" the liver and "cleansing" the blood. This addition to vitex therapy (1-3 droppersful in the morning each day) of the cooling and cleansing formulas usually brings excellent results. The base of the cleansing and cooling formula is as follows. It can be taken in tea or tincture form.

> *Burdock root (30%)*
> *Burdock seed (15%)*
> *Yellow Dock (15%)*
> *Oregon Grape root (20%)*
> *Red root (10%)*
> *Centaury (5%)*
>   *(or a small amount of gentian root if not available)*
> *Artichoke leaf (optional)*

Note: for flavor and sweetness, add fennel seed, orange peel, wintergreen leaf, chamomile, or mint (choose 1 or 2), and a little licorice. The herbs can also be ground up in a blender or (better) coffee grinder, the powder sieved through a fine screen, and then placed into "00" caps. Take 2-3 caps 2 x daily.

HEALTHY SKIN AND ACNE

*I*n order to insure success in the treatment of skin ailments like acne with vitex, it is advisable to support the vitex treatment with a diet high in natural fibers, reducing refined foods high in oils and sugar. Hydrotherapy and skin-brushing with a loofa or special skin brush is effective for increasing circulation to the skin to promote healing and remove excess waste products.

I recommend two forms of hydrotherapy. First, always finish a hot shower with a cold one, rinsing for at least 30 seconds to one minute. After experiencing the "glowing" feeling of the invigorating cold water, you may find it addictive. Second, splash areas affected with acne, such as the face, back or chest with hot water, or apply a hot compress for a few minutes. Then follow with a cold compress or splashes of cold water for up to a minute. This cycle can be repeated several times daily as needed. Because the skin has a very delicate "eco-system" all its own, flourishing with beneficial microorganisms and rich in protective fatty acids and other chemicals, it is important to pay special attention to its care. A good nutritious diet, exposure to lots of fresh air, exercise to increase blood circulation and the use of very mild soaps or no soap can increase skin vitality.

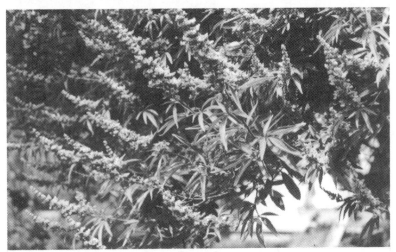

Figure 3

$\mathcal{U}$SING $\mathcal{U}$ITEX

How Long to Take Vitex?

Vitex should definitely be taken long-term for optimum effects. Clinical research shows that vitex may start working after about ten days, but for full benefit it should be taken up to six months or longer. For instance with PMS, it is likely that a positive result will be felt by the second period of menstruation. However, to create a permanent improvement, it may be necessary to take vitex for up to a year, and if the imbalance has been present for a long time (over 2 years), perhaps up to a year and a half.

It is important to remember that vitex is creating a fundamental change in the cyclic hormonal balance— and this takes time. Like herbs in general, vitex is a nourishing medicine that slowly, gently, and surely helps bring about a positive change in the body's delicate chemistry. In today's fast-paced society, we often want things to happen as quickly as possible, and so we are in the habit of relying on highly purified synthetic drugs (such as pure estrogen or even testosterone) which may produce immediate results—and, unfortunately, also unpleasant or even dangerous side effects. Again, herbs work in a different way. Instead of "shocking the body" into another set of symptoms or trying to force the body to change, blocking natural processes such as pain or fever, herbs work behind the scenes to harmonize, nourish, and restore balance in a gentle way. That's why many herbs, including vitex, have to be taken a long time to get the full results. This is not to say, however, that all herbs are completely safe to take in any way, at any dose. Some herbs are powerful medicinal agents and should be used with care.

Side Effects

Vitex has an unbeatable safety record: it has been used safely, with no reports of even moderate side effects, for over 2,000 years. In comparison, many modern drugs have unpleasant or outright dangerous side effects. Even aspirin, the virtual panacea of Western medicine, has had a dubious safety record over its period of use during the last century. There are numerous reports in the medical literature that show that its chronic use in therapeutic doses can lead to internal bleeding and liver disease.

Modern research confirms that vitex has no important side effects; thus European medical researchers have advocated the use of vitex and warned against over-use of synthetic hormones such as synthetic estrogen and progesterone, which do have possible side effects (Hahn et al, 1984). Nonetheless, it is not advisable to take vitex with progesterone or progesterone-containing medications (such as birth-control pills), because vitex may interfere with their activity (Madaus Agnolyt brochure). Also, it should be noted that during the first part of a treatment cycle using vitex, the length of the menstrual cycle may shorten or lengthen temporarily before it finally stabilizes (again, as stated in the Agnolyt brochure).

After 10 years of recommending vitex to friends and a few years of prescribing it in my clinic, I have no significant side effects to report. Other clinical herbalists from North America and Australia have advised me that they have seen an occasional skin rash, which goes away after a few days of discontinuing vitex use. Others have reported rare cases of reduced libido, which I have not personally seen. As with all herbal self-treatment, if you notice side effects, see a trained herbalist or health practitioner who can advise you about dose reduction or other useful herbs to use with vitex.

Dosage Information

Based on the Agnolyt therapeutic manual and clinical research, the average dosage of vitex should be 40 drops (1 dropperful) of the liquid extract or tincture, taken once a day in the morning on an empty stomach (about 1/2 hour before breakfast). If you prefer capsules, an equivalent dose would be about 3-4 capsules.

I have seen some herbalists use higher doses, up to 1 dropperful 3 times a day of liquid extract or tincture, especially for fibroid cysts. In this case 1 tablet of powdered extract should equal 1 dropperful of the liquid, depending on the relative concentrations. Depending on the severity of the hormonal imbalance, and the individual, my patients get the best results with 1-3 droppersful of the liquid tincture, 1-2 tablets containing powdered extract of vitex, or 4-6 capsules a day of simple powdered herb in capsules. When choosing a commercial vitex product, make sure to read the label to determine if it contains an extract, and if so, how much and how potent. If you are unsure about its potency, ask the supplement consultant where vitex is sold.

David Hoffmann recommends 2 ml (60 drops) of the liquid extract per day, and Annette Zeylstra, a British clinical herbalist with years of experience with vitex, says to take 3 ml (about 2 droppersful) before breakfast.

Synergistic Herbs

Synergistic herbs are herbs that may enhance the activity of the "lead" or main herbs in a formula, or reduce unwanted side effects. Table 5 lists some synergistic herbs for vitex.

For chronic health problems herbalists often recommend a formula or herbal combination which may contain as many as twelve herbs. With PMS, for example, it is probably best to combine vitex with other uterine tonic herbs such as blue cohosh, saw palmetto, or false unicorn root (star grass). For cramps, add cramp bark and wild yam, and so forth. Table 5 summarizes the use of some important herbs that work well with vitex. They can be found in most herb shops, both as single dry herbs and liquid tinctures, as well as components of numerous formulas for women's health. Average doses and common dose forms are given for reference, but the actual dose for your needs may vary.

TABLE 5. HERBS AND PHYTONUTRIENTS THAT WORK WELL WITH VITEX

Herb	Function	Dose
Wild Yam	helps reduce cramps; although advertised by some manufacturers for its progesterone-like properties, this effect has not been proven	1-3 dprsfl, 2 x day
Blue Cohosh	a nourishing, mildly stimulant uterine tonic; relieves pain	1-2 dprsfl, 2 x day
Dang Gui	nourishes the blood, tonifies female organs (dang gui is not hormonal)	3-9 gms/day in tea
Saw Palmetto	nourishes the female organs, relieves inflammation	3-9 gms/day in capsules
Dandelion	promotes milk flow, clears the liver	6-12 gms/day in tea
Black Cohosh	warms and stimulates the uterus, relieves pain, alleviates hot flashes, regulates estrogen	1-2 dprsfl 1-3 x day
Cramp Bark	helps relieve cramps	2-3 dprsfl 1-3 x day
Valerian	helps lessen cramps, calmative	2-3 dprsfl 1-3 x day
Cal. Poppy	relieves anxiety, calmative	2-3 dprsfl 1-3 x day
St. John's Wort	helps assuage mild depression	1-2 dprsfl 2-3 x day
Prickly Ash	very warming, helps direct herbs to the interior	3-9 gms/day in tea
Lavender	helps lift the spirits and strengthen the nerves	3-6 gms/day in tea

$\mathcal{V}$ITEX AND $\mathcal{C}$ONSTITUTIONAL $\mathcal{T}$YPES

Suppose two women take vitex, each of whom has heavy menstrual bleeding and other symptoms of hormonal imbalance. The treatment works splendidly with one woman, yet shows no results in the other. How can this be explained? (If you will recall, in the section on Modern Research it was noted that some researchers found that 35% of their patients showed no response to vitex).

Each of us has a unique biochemical and physical makeup and responds to our environment in different ways. All of our habits and genetic tendencies combined make up our *constitution*, or our body's pattern of responding to its environment. Ancient systems of medicine such as Traditional Chinese Medicine and Ayurveda (the healing system of India), recognize several different constitutional types and understand that herbal and other holistic treatments have to be geared differently for each constitutional type. What works for one person doesn't necessarily work for another of a different constitutional type. Western medicine used to have a concept of constitutional types, but for the most part this understanding disappeared with the onset of the current industrial and scientific model of medicine. However, this is rapidly changing, through the influence of our shrinking world and individuals becoming more receptive to the healing way of the heart and the spirit.

Now if a person (say, the woman above who didn't benefit from vitex) has what is called a "weakened" constitution—perhaps she has an underlying delicate genetic heritage which has been aggravated by less than ideal living habits—then she will probably not enjoy the full effects of vitex immediately. First she needs to re-build her energy reserves and regain overall balance by taking "tonic herbs" along with vitex. For instance, if her immune system is weak—as is often the case with people who have been under stress for many years, or have eaten mostly processed foods, or have received a long course of treatment with antibiotics or steroids such as cortisone—then immune tonics or adrenal tonics would be recommended along with vitex and all the necessary changes in diet and lifestyle. Without such a holistic program, some women (about 35%, according to the experiment in question) will not feel any positive results from taking vitex.

Now you may be wondering how to tell whether you or someone you know has a weakened constitution. One sure sign is if, along with symptoms of PMS or hormonal imbalance, other symptoms such as environmental sensitivity, allergies, chronic fatigue, or chronic candida overgrowth are also present. Table 6 gives information about other herbs or herbal formulas to add when there is constitutional weakness or adrenal fatigue.

TABLE 6. SUPPORTING HERBS FOR STRESS AND CONSTITUTIONAL FACTORS

Formulas or single Herbs

Symptoms	Situation	to add to Vitex
Low energy, dizziness, that 'worn-our' feeling due to overwork and stress	stressful environment, general stress, chronic fatigue	add eleuthero, schizandra, ashwaganda, American ginseng, adrenal support formula
Allergies (to food, environmental factors), chronic infections	poor nutrition, long-term stress, environmental toxicity (pesticide poisoning, heavy metal poisoning, etc.)	add astragalus, ligustrum, reishi, (immune tonics); warming foods such as yams, barley; and superfoods such as spirulina, etc.
Short-term infection of bladder (cystitis)	burning upon urination, cloudy urine	drink cranberry juice; add herbs such as pipsissewa, usnea, saw palmetto, sandalwood every 3 hours
Fatigue, pale face, tongue, anemia	possible blood deficiency	1 serving of steamed greens/day; other chlorophyll-rich foods such as barley greens powder or spirulina; blood-tonic herbs such as nettles, yellow dock, or dang gui; and digestive bitters in liquid form before meals

*For candidiasis, try echinacea in 10-day cycles (up to 3), or 10 drops of the liquid extract once or twice a day for up to 6 months. Add black walnut in capsule or liquid extract and pau d'arco as anti-fungals, along with the "deep immune" builders mentioned above.

There are, of course, many other constitutional types besides just "weakened constitution," but a full discussion of all of them is beyond the scope of this work. For further reading on this fascinating subject, as well as a basic explanation of Traditional Chinese Medicine and Ayurvedic Medicine, I recommend several books in the reading list at the end of this booklet.

In the case where symptoms of PMS or menstrual irregularities are present (for example, heavy bleeding, cramping, and depression which disappear at the onset of bleeding), then tonic herbs for the sexual organs may be called for, such as blue cohosh, false unicorn root, and dang gui, among others (see the section on Synergistic Herbs for more). Vitex as a single remedy can provide excellent results where only female hormonal imbalances are concerned—and nothing else—though in many other situations herbs often work better in combination.

$\mathcal{S}$HOPPING FOR $\mathcal{V}$ITEX $\mathcal{P}$RODUCTS

Quality considerations

To be effective, the quality of a given herbal product should be considered carefully. There are two main factors to look at when determining the quality of an herbal product:

1) How old the product is and the form of the product (tincture, powder, etc.)
2) The quality of the original herb that makes up the product

To determine how old an herbal product is, look at the manufacture or the "pull" (expiration) date on the bottle. Try not to buy a tincture or liquid product that is over 3 years old, or capsules that are more than 1 1/2 years old (ideally capsules should be under 1 year old). If there is no date of any kind on the bottle, call the manufacturer and ask how long ago the herb was bottled. Of course, for this the manufacturer will need the lot number—and if that isn't on the bottle either, you really don't want the product.

To determine the quality of an herb, take the whole herb (or the powder from a capsule), spread it on the palm of your hand, and rub it back and forth with your thumb, as you cup the hand containing the herb. This process should release the volatile oils in the herb. Now smell the herb—if it does not have a resinous, aromatic smell, or if it smells moldy, reject the bottle. Don't feel like you're being too "picky" by returning the bottle to the store and telling the store owner; this sort of consumer response is crucial to help interest manufacturers in paying more attention to the quality of the herbs they sell. There are some very good herbal products out there—and some that aren't so good. By choosing carefully you can purchase the best possible product and help raise the general quality of herbal products on the market.

$\mathcal{D}$OSE FORMS: LIQUIDS, POWDERS, OR TEA?

Powders

Powdered herbs can be found in tablet form or in capsules. Powders are simply ground-up herb (in the case of vitex, it is the seeds that are powdered). The good thing about powders is that they are not processed in any way (except powdering), and products made from powder are usually cost-effective. But on the down side, powdered products usually have a reduced shelf-life (use within one year of manufacturing), and more of a powdered product needs to be taken in order to get a good dose. For instance, 1 dropperful of the liquid extract usually equals about 3 capsules of powder, depending on the quality of the herb.

Liquid Extracts

In Europe, the most common products containing vitex are liquid and powdered extracts. Agnolyt, the product on which most scientific research on vitex has been performed, is a liquid extract.

Another name for a liquid extract is a *tincture*. In the case of vitex, liquid extracts are made by grinding the whole seed into powder and then soaking the powder in a solvent of grain alcohol and water for several weeks. The solvent "absorbs" and concentrates the active constituents of the herb, and then the remaining solids (from the powder) can be pressed and filtered out. The resulting tincture, or liquid extract, is an excellent medicine, because the alcohol acts as a carrier, slightly stimulates digestion and assimilation, and is a very good preservative. Liquid extracts should hold their active properties for up to three years, provided they are stored in a cool place out of the direct sunlight.

The amount of alcohol in a dose of herbal extract (usually about 40 drops, or one dropperful) is very small. When one dropperful of tincture is diluted in a small glass of juice or water, the final percentage of alcohol in the mixture becomes tiny—less than 0.1%. There may be more ethyl alcohol in a ripe banana! Nonetheless, if you are opposed to taking even this small amount of alcohol, try some of the other dose forms discussed below.

Another type of liquid extract becoming available is called a *glycerite*, which is made from glycerin derived from either animal or vegetable sources. There are several things to be aware of about glycerites. First, you may want to ask the manufacturer of your product whether it contains animal or vegetable glycerin. Second, glycerin can be irritating (much as is alcohol) and drying to the throat and digestive tract (unlike alcohol), so it is best to take in water. A third possible drawback with glycerites is that they may not be as concentrated as tinctures. To make a glycerite, first the herbs have to be extracted in alcohol, then the alcohol is removed by heating (hopefully as little as possible and under vacuum), and finally the glycerin added. At this point, all the active constituents that were dissolved in the alcohol may not go into solution in the glycerin, because glycerin has different properties as a solvent than alcohol (Wood and Remington, 1894). Thus a one-ounce bottle of a glycerite may be weaker than a comparable bottle of alcohol-based tincture. In the case of vitex, the active constituents are not entirely known, but they may be resinoid compounds or flavonoids, both of which are more soluble in alcohol than in glycerin.

Powdered Extracts

Powdered extracts are made by taking the liquid extract one step further. The liquid is "spray-dried" under a flash of hot air into a vacuum. This process dries the liquid extract to a powder that has been stripped of the ingredients that are not medicinally important (such as the fiber, fatty oil, and starch). The resulting powder is then pressed into tablets or packed into capsules which, like the liquid extract, have been "pre-digested" and are easily and quickly assimilated by the body.

Tea

If you want to make your own homemade tea or capsules—which can be just as effective as the other dose forms, provided the herb you use is fresh and of good quality—you can buy vitex in bulk at an herb or health-food store. Fortunately, the shelf-life of whole vitex is quite long because the fruits, which are the parts of the plant used in herbal medicine, are covered with a hard shell. However, be aware of the fact that as soon as the fruits are ground into powder, oxygen immediately starts to react with and destroy the plant's active chemical substances. Thus it is always best to buy the bulk herb in its whole state (complete fruits) whenever possible and then to grind it as needed for tea or to make capsules. In the case of vitex fruits, the taste is a little spicy and bitter, so try mixing them with chamomile, ginger, and a little licorice to enhance the flavor. The medicinal activity will not be adversely affected.

Whatever form of vitex you choose to take—whether a liquid glycerite or alcohol-based extract, powdered herb in capsules or powdered extract in capsules or tablets, or even your own homemade tea—is really an individual preference. The most important thing is to use a high-quality herb or herbal product that is not too old.

Finally, whenever possible, choose a product that is organically-grown (look for the label that says **certified organically-grown**). Organic farming supports the natural growth-cycle of plants, does not add to our planet's pollution, and preserves the wild populations of plants which are now increasingly being over-harvested to make herbal medicines. In the case of vitex, however, organically-grown fruits are not available yet. Therefore, much of the herb is harvested from the wild in southern

Europe. Just look for the fruits to be aromatic (they should have a distinct, resinous odor when crushed) and free from dirt or a moldy smell.

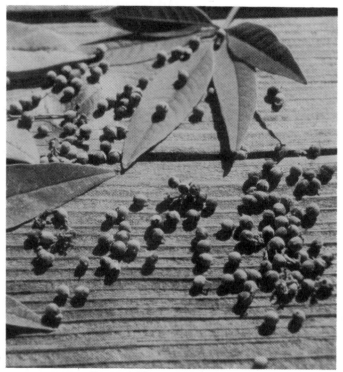

Figure 4. Vitex seeds and leaves

Clinical Experience of Modern Herbalists

Annette Zeylstra

Annette Zeylstra, a medical herbalist from England, is a practitoner specializing in women's health issues with years of experience with vitex. I first learned of the usefulness and popularity of vitex in 1985 from Ms. Zeylstra. She considers vitex a standard treatment for PMS and menopause and gives 35 drop doses of the liquid extract daily before breakfast.

David Hoffmann

David Hoffmann, a well-trained and highly experienced English medical herbalist and author of *The Holistic Herbal*, reports that the most important use of vitex in England is for treating symptoms of menopause, and that this is the *only* female health situation in which he uses vitex by itself. For relieving symptoms such as hot flashes, he claims good results can be obtained after two or three months of taking 2 ml (65 drops) of vitex a day. One of the main points that Hoffmann stresses is the need to use vitex in combination with other tonifying herbs that strengthen the female organs, such as blue cohosh and false unicorn root (star grass or *Chamaelirium luteum*). He finds this to be especially true with PMS.

David also emphasizes that vitex should be taken long-term, up to six months, but that improvements can be seen sometimes within two or three weeks. The other herbs he likes to combine vitex with are St. John's wort (*Hypericum perforatum*), to help counteract the symptoms of depression which often accompany PMS and menopause; and skullcap, to help alleviate cramps.

Brenda Jackson, Nurse Practitioner, Herbalist

Brenda Jackson, a nurse practitioner who uses herbs and other natural methods in her practice, says that at least 70% of the women she works with have some kind of hormonally-based imbalance. She has used vitex in practice for about six years in hundreds of patients, mostly for helping with PMS, menopause, fibroids, and occasionally endometriosis.

She nearly always mixes the vitex with 3-5 additional herbs, depending on the person and the situation. For PMS she combines vitex with 3-5 additional herbs, such as licorice, sarsaparilla, and wild yam, depending on the person and the situation. She often adds lymphatic or diuretic herbs if applicable. For menopause, she adds more black or blue cohosh, licorice, or other estrogenic herbs to the formula.

Ms. Jackson prefers to give a substantial dose of the liquid extract, usually 1 tsp. of the combination 3 times daily. She often gets a response in one month, sometimes by the second or third month. She finds that three months is a good treatment period, and after following up with many of her patients, she commonly finds lasting effects. If a woman does not respond within three months, she changes the formula, adding other herbs, and sometimes refers the patient for acupuncture treatments. She feels thyroid imbalance is fairly common in these cases. Ms. Jackson has seen easing of symptoms in endometriosis and has had success with fibroids—especially ones that are on the external wall (less positive results with internal ones).

Holly Guzman, Licensed Acupuncturist

When I recommend vitex, I initially use it during the second half of the menstrual cycle, up until bleeding is expected. Some women are more quickly effected by vitex, and if their progesterone levels increase rapidly within one cycle, then this is the best timing. If changes are not obvious within this two-week trial, then daily usage can begin and be continued over six months. After a woman is no longer ovulating, even randomly, the vitex is no longer my herb of choice, as its stimulus to the ovaries and corpus luteum is not effectual. I then recommend menopausal support with herbs and foods that assist the adrenals or contain phytosterols to assist endocrine balance, such as American ginseng and soybean; herbs that help with mineral balance for the bones, such as nettles; and/or herbs that support the heart, such as motherwort and hawthorn.

Lois Johnson, M.D.

Vitex is the most important herb I use for women's health issues. It is appropriate for the whole range of diseases related to hormonal imbalance from PMS and dysmenorrhea to endometriosis and menopause.

My Own Experience

I have seen one case in which a fibroid cyst was successfully treated with vitex, and received reports from several other women who have read this book and had success with their fibroids after taking vitex. Some have seen reductions in size in the fibroids after several months, and a few told me the fibroids seemed to disappear. Vitex has to be taken for at least 4-6 months. The first woman mentioned was 38 and had extremely heavy bleeding combined with headache, cramps, and malaise during menstruation. The symptoms were so severe that she often had to take a day or two off of work during her period. This situation continued over a period of at least ten years, and then she began to take a formula consisting of vitex (50%), black and blue cohosh (20%), lavender (10%), dandelion (10%), and prickly ash (10%). She took 3 or 4 droppersful a day for 4 months. During the treatment she felt like the month-to-month symptoms were somewhat better, and for a few months the bleeding was not as heavy. After two months, however, she began to spot lightly between menstrual periods, and after four months, she began to experience very heavy bleeding. At this point she went to a medical doctor, and a bloody mass was eliminated. From that moment on, she started to get better: her periods became lighter and more normal, and the other symptom gradually disappeared. After several years she is still much better.

I have seen other cases where a similar blend of vitex and other herbs was used for psychological disturbances which began before and disappeared with the onset of the menstrual period. In these cases, there was a long-term improvement in emotional ups and downs.

$\mathcal{A}$PPENDIX A

$\mathcal{B}$OTANY

Vitex (*agnus castus*) is a genus from the Verbenaceae family and consists of about 60 species in the tropics and subtropics in both hemispheres. It grows from the size of a shrub to that of a small tree (3-9 feet tall), mostly in the area from the Mediterranean to western Asia, though I have seen vitex trees grow up to 20 feet tall in California. The bark is white-felted, the opposite leaves are palmately compound with 5-7 leaflets, and the long spires of pale lilac- or rose- colored flowers are in interrupted spikes, corolla two-lipped, 6-9 mm long. The fruits (which are the parts used medicinally) are small, hard, reddish-black drupes with a persistent calyx (Rehder, 1927; Polunin, 1987). Vitex is often found growing next to streams, for it loves water, but I have also seen it growing in very dry spots on the Greek islands.

$\mathcal{C}$HEMISTRY

The three main fractions of the vitex's fruit include: essential oil; two iridoid glycosides, aucubin and agnuside; fixed fatty oil; and the flavone, casticin (Steinegger, 1988). Three further minor flavonoids were recently characterized as 3,6,7,4'-tetramethyl ether of 6-hydroxykaempferol, the 3,6,7-tri-Me ether of 6-hyroxykaempferol, and the 3,6,7-tri-Me ether of quercetagetin (Wollenweber, 1983).

The dried fruits contain about 0.5 to 1.22% essential oil, which is mainly composed of cineol (25.2%), alpha- and beta- pinene (39.7%), and limonene (14.8%) (Mishurova, 1986). The leaves, which are also used in folk-medicine, contain: 3 iridoid glycosides, aucubin, agnuside, and eurostoside; (Goerler, 1985) the flavonoids homo-orientin and luteolin-7-glucoside; and 0.76 to 0.82% essential oil (Mishurova, 1986).

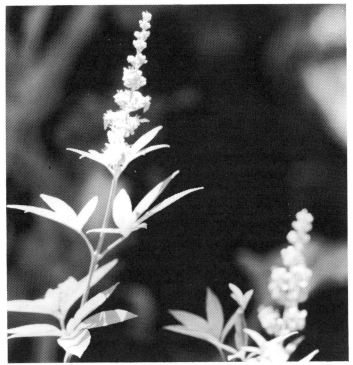

Figure 5

𝒫HARMACOLOGY

Dr. Gerhard Madaus began laboratory experiments with vitex in the 1930s and found it to have a "strong corpus-luteum" effect. In several case histories, he reported that the onset of menstruation was sometimes delayed for a few days after administration of vitex, for which the herb rosemary was an effective antidote, inducing menstrual flow immediately.

In 1954, Probst and Roth used vitex successfully to treat hyper- and polymenorrhea. Based on earlier experiments showing a progesteronic effect, researchers assumed that vitex contained a progesterone-like substance. However, Buchholz, Koch, Uebel, and Haller then found in experiments on animals that vitex indirectly stimulates the production of progesterone through the anterior lobe of the pituitary gland, inducing luteinization (Hahn, 1984).

Throughout the 1950s and 1960s, clinical trials showed that vitex was effective in treating menstrual difficulties as well as acne and constipation due to increased estrogen levels, and recent findings confirm that vitex helps restore a normal estrogen-to-progesterone balance (Hahn, 1984). Research also shows that vitex increases lactation (again through pituitary activation), and that it has an anti-bacterial effect (Mishurova, 1986; De Capite, 1967).

According to the Agnolyt detail manual (supplied by Madaus), vitex's major methods of activity can be summarized as follows:

1. The primary site of activity is the anterior lobe of the pituitary gland.

2. It inhibits follicle-stimulating hormone (FSH).
3. It increases secretion of luteinising hormone (LH).
4. It increases secretion of luteotropic hormone (LTH); that is, it stimulates the formation of the corpus luteum.

*P*HARMACOGNOSY

By far the most common part of vitex sold in the herb trade is the small (5 mm), dry fruits, containing 4 seeds. These seeds are gray-black, taste slightly peppery (they are called "monk's pepper" in Germany), and are resinous when chewed. Under the microscope, the exocarp (shell) is covered with short glandular hairs. The fruits should not taste musty or moldy and should not have too much dirt, rocks, or twigs mixed in.

Chemically, vitex can be standardized to the essential oil. The dried fruits should contain between 0.4 and 0.5% total essential oil (List, 1973).

*P*HARMACY

In Germany, the liquid extract or tincture of vitex is usually made with 1 part of the dried fruits to 10 parts of 95% ethanol (grain alcohol). This makes a "homeopathic mother tincture," which is then further diluted for other homeopathic remedies.

Manufacturers in the United States may make the liquid extract at 1 part fruit to 5 parts menstruum (1:5), or up to 1:4, which usually means that there is much more extracted matter (or solids) in the finished tincture (Steinegger, 1988), Whether this means that the preparation will be stronger depends on one's philosophy. Many American herbalists feel that the more solids, the stronger the medicine, and many Europeans feel that a weaker "mother tincture" may be stronger. This latter philosophy follows the homeopathic principal that "like cures like," and highly diluted extracts are stronger, energetically, than when less diluted.

CULTIVATION

There are two varieties of *Vitex agnus castus*: alba (white lilac chaste tree), and latifolia (hardy lilac chaste tree) (Kelsey, 1942). I have commonly seen two forms of vitex—one seems to grow into a small tree, while the other remains a bush, but the difference may be accounted for by environmental conditions, not genetic variation. It is possible to find vitex plants at the nursery, or you can order one.

Vitex plants like a good amount of water. I had one plant which was just straggling along until I accidentally left it under a leaky faucet. The amount of growth it put on under that faucet was amazing! Since then I've been giving all of my vitex plants a great deal more water— with the result that they now do much better. Remember that the Romans likened vitex to *Salix*, the willow, another group of water-loving plants.

Vitex plants are hardy and will lose their leaves in the winter. However, the spring growth is tender to a late frost, so the young plants should be covered with straw or mulch in cold areas.

To propagate the plants, put the cuttings in a light, well-drained soil early in the spring, before the buds begin to swell. Water them frequently and they will take root. Layering also works well with vitex (Green, 1823), but with this technique you should be careful when bending the branches to the ground, otherwise they may split. Then barely cover the branches with dirt, water them in dry weather, and they should take root in one year. Set the cuttings out in March, but be careful of frost. The plants tend to sucker, so it is good to trim the shrub and focus its energy on the top flowering and fruiting shoots.

Vitex has beautiful sprays of white and lilac-to-blue colored flowers in late summer or early fall. They make an excellent ornamental, because they bloom when most other plants don't.

If you're trying to grow the plants for the seed, keep in mind that vitex will probably not seed in a cool coastal climate. They require hot summers. I have not been able to get mine to fruit in Santa Cruz, but I have friends who have gotten good crops from individual plants in southern Oregon, where it is much hotter in the summer. Green, in his famous *Universal Herbal*, mentions that vitex will not fruit or even finish flowering in England during a particularly cold year.

$\mathcal{A}$PPENDIX B

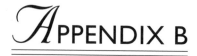

$\mathcal{V}$ITEX VERSUS SYNTHETIC HORMONE THERAPY

With so many options in the treatment of female cyclic disorders, it is crucial to carefully evaluate the choices of therapy. In our current pharmacy, we are bombarded by the selections and controversies surrounding natural and synthetic medicines. This chapter will review the use of vitex versus synthetically derived hormones.

The Hormone Therapy Revolution

Prior to this century, phytomedicines were the only remedies available for the treatment of disease. However, with the development of pharmaceuticals came a revolution of highly purified and concentrated synthetic drugs. Some of the first synthetic progesterones were prepared in the 1930s with extracts from the Mexican Wild Yam. These new drugs, for the first time, provided doctors the ability to control the body's internal chemistry. With the success of synthetic drugs many well-proven natural remedies were forgotten.

The introduction of synthetic drugs into the pharmacopeia marked a significant change in the direction of healthcare throughout the Western World. With this new technology, doctors learned to control the natural hormone balance, as shown by the effects of birth control pills. Physicians also utilize synthetic hormones to treat a variety of disorders such as PMS, premenopausal symptoms, CLI, hyperprolactinemia, and a host of uterine and bleeding disorders.

A variety of synthetic hormone preparations have been developed for the treatment of specific cyclic disorders. These drugs fall under two main divisions, those which are progesterone-like (progestins) and those estrogen-like (estrogens). A prescription to one of these treatments is dependent upon the diagnosed deficiency, age, and health history. In addition, it is important to recognize the method of drug delivery because some hormones may be taken dermally (topical application to the skin), intravenously, or via suppositories. Table 7 lists common cyclic disorders, their corresponding hormone treatments and side effects.

Effects of Hormone Therapy

During the sixty years since its introduction, hormone replacement therapy has brought successful treatments as well as a host of problems. The original enthusiasm experienced by physicians for these powerful drugs has drastically changed in recent years as more information about their true effects has surfaced. Current debate in the medical community centers around concern for safety and long-term side effects, which are well documented by hundreds of clinical studies and trials by pharmaceuticals. Commonly reported side effects are nausea, breast tenderness, and retention of sodium and water which may irritate cardiac and kidney function. More extreme, though less common, ones include impairment of ovaries, formation of cysts, related emotional changes and depression, weight gain, cancer, cardiovascular diseases, and various sexual disorders (Attelmann

TABLE 7: COMMONLY PRESCRIBED SYNTHETIC HORMONE PREPARATIONS BY MEDICAL DOCTORS

Cyclic Disorder	Prescribed Hormone	Influence	Side Effects
Menopause without hysterectomy**	Combination of estrogens* and progestins. Premerin is the most commonly prescribed synthetic conjugated estrogen and Provera, for progesterone. Progestin should be added on calendar days 1 to 12. Sequential therapy of progestins is safer than continuous	The goal of the treatment is to alleviate symptoms, such as hot flashes, urogenital atrophy, osteoporosis, and possibly, coronary heart disease. Treatment should also improve libido, mood, and sleep.	Nausea, mastaigia, menstrual bleeding, might increase necessity for surgery, uterine and breast cancer, thromboembolic disease, stomach irritation, edema of the feet and lower legs, hypertension and gallstones.
Menopause with a hysterectomy**	Estrogens (Premerin).* Progestins are not recommended for women without an intact uterus.	The goal of the treatment is to alleviate symptoms, such as hot flashes, urogenital atrophy, osteoporosis, and possibly, coronary heart disease. Treatment should also improve libido, mood, and sleep.	Nausea, fullness and tenderness of breast, Increases levels of HDL cholesterol. Might increase risk of uterine and breast cancer, thromboembolic disease, hypertension, stomach irritation, edema of the feet and lower legs, and gallstones.
PMS**	Oral contraceptives estrogen/progesterone combination (eg. Ortho-novum 1/35, norethindone and mestranol, norgesterel and ethinyl estradiol, norethindone and ethinyl estradiol). Natural progesterone or pyridoxine/spironolactone.	The goal is to relieve symptoms of PMS. Contraceptives are effective in removing acne from premenstrual acne. Previous medical protocols recommend oral contraceptives. Today, however, they are occasionally used for this purpose.	Undesirable side effects develop in at least 25% of patients on oral contraceptives. Short-term effects include nausea, headache, acne, stomach pain, and weight gain. Long-term side effects include cardiovascular diseases, liver cancer, stroke, uterine problems, and hypertension.

(Table 7 continued on page 45)

Table 7, continued

Cyclic Disorder	Prescribed Hormone	Influence	Side Effects
Dysmenorrhea (painful menstruation)	Oral contraceptives (eg. Ortho-novum 1/35, norethindone and mestranol, norgesterel and ethinyl estradiol, norethindone and ethinyl estradiol).	Oral contraceptives are very effective; however, most cases can be treated without hormones. Prostaglandin synthetase inhibitors, such phenylproplonic acid derivatives (ibuprofen), acetic acid derivatives and fenamates are very effective.	Undesirable side effects develop in at least 25% of patients on oral contraceptives. Short-term effects include nausea, headache, acne, stomach pain, and weight gain. Long-term use side effects include cardiovascular disease, liver cancer, stroke, uterine problems, and hypertension.
Endometriosis**	Danazol, Enovid, Depo-Provera (progestogens). Oral contraceptives, are used in 40% of patients, the most common drug regimen.	The treatment goal is to create a state of pseudopregnancy/menopause in order to stop growth of the endometrial wall.	Danazol–decrease in breast size, irregular menstrual periods, weight gain, slight possibility of vaginal dryness and itching. Patient may be photosensitive. Oral contraceptives–nausea, headache, acne, stomach pain, and weight gain. Potential for cardiovascular diseases, liver cancer, and stroke.
Amenorrhea	Clomiphene citrate (Clomid)	The goal is to initiate menstrual bleeding; Clomiphene is a fertility medicine to help women become pregnant.	Bloating stomach or pelvic pain, hot flashes. This medicine is usually used for a short period of time, so long-term side effects are not of major concern.

* Estrogen should be used continuously without interruption.

**Estrogen contraindicated to individuals with a history of breast or endometrial cancers

& Bends, 1972). *The Complete Drug Reference*, a prescription resource guide, mentions severe side effects and concerns about the use of progestins which include blood clots, heart attacks, strokes, liver disease and cancer, problems with the eyes, discharge from the breast, stomach pain, skin rash or itching, mental depression, and anemia (*Complete Drug Reference*, 1993).

In addition, there is a concern that long-term hormone therapy may be dangerous. Not only does the patient run the risk of temporary side effects, but the consistent use of synthetics has been known to further health complications. Years of continuous treatment may permanently damage the hypothalamus and pituitary glands, desensitizing the receptors crucial for hormone regulation (Probst, 1954).

The very nature of synthetic hormones makes them a center of concern. Synthetic hormones have a different molecular structure from the natural estrogens and progesterone secreted by the body. Many of the drugs are more potent and have a greater binding affinity for estrogen and progesterone receptors. In addition, some of the drugs may target tissues and organs that are not normally acted upon by the natural hormones. The liver, the organ responsible for breaking down and recycling the body's hormones, may have difficulty recognizing and processing synthetic hormones. One significant side effect of long term hormone replacement therapy is liver cancer and disease.

What are the Alternatives?

There are a vast number of holistic oriented alternative therapies to supersede the conventional hormone replacement therapy. In fact, many of these therapeutic options don't even require the use of botanical medicines. Changes in lifestyle and diet, moderate exercise, stress reduction and relaxation practices (yoga and meditation), and support groups, are just to name a few. I have found that many women will experience a remarkable change following the above mentioned options. When we become caught up in the stressors of modern society, eating highly processed nutrient poor foods and being exposed to stress in the work place or at home, we lose the ability to maintain a hormonal balance. Positive lifestyle changes should be a crucial part of any therapy for hormonal and menstrual imbalances. Getting back in touch with ourselves, finding the optimum balance between health and work, family and friends is the ultimate goal of therapy.

There are, without a doubt, individuals with hormone imbalances who will require a more potent therapy. Every body is unique and some women will find great value in searching out a direct therapy to stimulate the synthesis of sex hormones. For these individuals, there are several herbal preparations to stimulate the female endocrine system. Long term use of vitex in combination with dang gui, rehmannia, black cohosh, and wild yam will stimulate the replacement of the sex hormones (see previous sections on herbs for menopause).

A beautiful aspect in the practice of medicine is the degree of variation evident within every human body. Some women may invest a great deal of energy into their bodies—exercising regularly, eating a nutritious organic diet, and striving to eliminate stress, and yet they may still suffer from a hormone imbalance; while others may seldom exercise, eat foods low in nutrition, and mildly suffer from a hormone imbalance (this may be due to different constitutional types). Overall, however, these cases are rare. It is evident that placing value on the quality of life corresponds directly to our sense of well being. There is no sure method to prevent imbalance and disease. In spite of that, investing energy into maintaining a healthy body and mind will bring about an immediate sense of control, strength, and balance, and contribute towards prevention of illness.

The following reviews preventive measures and herbal treatments for hormone imbalances.

Dietary Recommendations — A recommended diet centers around complex carbohydrates, including whole grains, legumes, vegetables, and fruits. Avoid polyunsaturated vegetable oils and foods that are high in sugar and alcohol because they promote reactive hypoglycemia, a major source of PMS symptoms. Women suffering from edema should avoid salt to reduce fluid retention. Finally, women should not consume chocolate or beverages with caffeine, because these foods will increase tension and irritability.

Vitamin and Mineral Supplements — Vitamin B6 and mineral supplements, particularly antioxidants and magnesium in relatively high doses, are recommended.

Exercise Program — A regular exercise program, such as swimming, aerobics, and/or walking, is recommended to decrease depression, anxiety, and fluid retention. There are several studies documenting the positive hormonal effects of exercise in women.

Stress Maintenance Program — A relaxation program including yoga and meditation may help calm the nerves.

Herbal Treatment — There are many botanical approaches towards the treatment of PMS. Some of the treatments, such as vitex, focus on the root cause of PMS through regulating the synthesis of hormones by the hypothalamus-pituitary axis. Other herbs, such as cramp bark or raspberry leaf, are prescribed to specifically treat symptoms. A recommended herbal treatment would combine both methods—providing the patient first with immediate symptomatic relief; and second, a long-term formula for restoring and building health.

Long-term herbal therapy — A vitex formula with the addition of dang gui, rehmannia root, codonopsis, nettles, and dandelion may be taken over a period of several months.

An Integrative Comparison

Although their approaches may differ widely, the ultimate goal of both conventional and herbal medicine is to remove the disorder with minimal side effects. This task, however, is particularly challenging in the treatment of female cyclic disorders. Because the hormone system is not isolated to a particular organ, the effects of treatment may be experienced throughout the entire body.

Conventional medicine approaches most of these conditions with the administration of synthetic hormones. The reasoning behind this treatment is to mimic or intensify the biological effects of the body's natural hormones (*AMA Drug Evaluations*, 1983). In many situations, hormone therapy is fast-acting and provides symptomatic relief. For instance, estrogen replacement therapy is extremely effective in providing relief from hot flashes and other menopausal symptoms. However, the question remains as to whether these drugs are safe for long-term treatment of the disorder. At this point in time, the answer is unclear. It has been shown that many of these synthetic drugs are poorly tolerated by the body and are accompanied by a variety of side effects (see Table 7 for overview of drug side effects). Since hormone replacement therapy must be given on a long-term basis for menopause, there are a potential host of problems that may be created from years of continual use. On the other hand, there are many benefits from hormone replacement therapy. For example, estrogen and progesterone replacement therapy in menopausal patients alleviates hot flashes, urogenital atrophy, osteoporosis, and possibly coronary heart diseases, in addition to improvement in sexual response, mood, sleep, and memory (Utian, 1990). All in all, the medical community is still undecided in their response to hormone replacement therapy. Research will continue in the years ahead and will be costly in terms of general health and dollars.

Vitex, on the other hand, is an effective therapy with excellent tolerance and mild action. Unlike synthetics, vitex is not a hormone. Vitex acts to solve the disorder through biological regulation. This presents a major advantage in therapeutic use for certain gynecological conditions which cannot accept sex hormones. Additionally, vitex does not cause the side effects often experienced with hormone therapy. Toxicological analysis and clinical studies of women's tolerance of vitex have not reported any significant side effects (Amman, 1982).

The success of therapy with vitex is remarkable. Most recent clinical studies report an average success rate of 85% (Feldmann, 1995; Peters-Welte, 1994; Amberg,

1994; Milewicz, 1993; Loch, 1991; Coeugniet, 1986).
Vitex improves symptoms within several weeks to
months, depending upon the condition. Since there are
no contraindications, vitex may also be used with synthetic hormone therapy (Foster, 1994). It is also the
optimum choice of therapy if the patient desires a pregnancy (Amman, 1982). (See Table 8 for overall benefits
and supporting use of vitex).

Nonetheless, there are certain situations in which the
use of synthetic hormones is desirable. Cases of severe
ovarian dysfunction require treatment with synthetics.
For example, the only treatment option for advanced
corpus luteum insufficiency is progesterone and/or
estrogen. However, if the patient had diagnosed the
condition early, then synthetics might not have been
necessary. Therapy with vitex would have no effect in
such advanced conditions.

In the treatment of cyclic disorders, a proper diagnosis
is critical. The type of condition, severity of symptoms,
and personal health history will dictate the appropriate
treatment. Mild conditions will usually respond favorably
to vitex treatment, while advanced cases may require
hormone replacement therapy. Early diagnosis as well as
good health practices (diet and exercise) will optimize
success with vitex.

A Professional Opinion

Today, medical experts generally caution against
indiscriminate use of highly potent hormone preparations. With growing concern regarding the tolerance of
hormones, natural medicines are becoming an accepted
alternative treatment. Principally, the German medical
community is leading the integration of vitex into main-
stream medicine. Almost all clinical studies on vitex have

TABLE 8: SUMMARY SUPPORTING THE USE OF VITEX: "THE VITEX TOP TEN"

1. Vitex is a sensible and proven alternative to hormone replacement therapy.

2. Vitex acts to normalize the hormone imbalance through the pituitary gland, correcting the problem at the source.

3. The action of vitex is indirect because the herb is not an actual hormone. Therefore, effects of vitex therapy are mild and can occur over an extended period.

4. Vitex therapy has few side effects, with as low as 1-2% of cases reporting problems. Alternately, synthetic hormone therapy may produce effects with serious complications.

5. Vitex is taken orally, while some synthetic hormones require rectal/vaginal suppositories, topical administration [patches can cause skin irritation and are often inconvenient], or intravenous injection for delivery.

6. Vitex may be taken continuously, independent of the menstrual cycle.

7. Vitex aids in the production of breast milk. In contrast, progesterone and estrogen therapy must be discontinued during breastfeeding.

8. Vitex therapy for mild disorders can often be terminated several months after symptoms disappear. On the contrary, synthetic hormones sometimes require long-term treatment.

9. Vitex carries the experiences and wisdom of many generations and cultures. Additionally, vitex is supported by modern clinical trials. On the other hand, synthetic hormones are lacking any history beyond sixty years of clinical application.

10. The cost of hormone replacement therapy is substantially higher than vitex. The cost of standardized extract tablets is approximately nine dollars per month, or seven dollars per month for liquids or formulas containing vitex. One month of continuous conjugated estrogen (Premarin) and medroxyprogesterone (Provera) is approximately thirty-one dollars per month. "Natural" progesterone and estradiol treatment is approximately twenty-five dollars per month. This figure depends upon the rates at your local pharmacy.

been performed by German physicians. Table 9 summarizes the contribution by these physicians and their opinions concerning synthetic hormone treatment and vitex.

TABLE 9: RECOMMENDATIONS FROM MEDICAL DOCTORS

Clinical Study Overview	Comments on Synthetic Hormone vs. Vitex Treatment	Physicians
This well-planned study observed the effectiveness and tolerance for the treatment of PMS with vitex. 551 patients participated over 4 months.	". . . patients are now more critical toward hormonal medication and prefer herbal preparations which, with milder action, produce fewer side effects. The results of the study showed that a high percentage of women can be best treated over an extended period with vitex, with almost no side effects. . . . The effectiveness of the preparation shows that Agnolyt (vitex) should be used as a continuous preparation whenever a specific, but mild therapy for regulatory disorders of the menstrual cycle is clearly indicated."	Dr. Peter-Welle (1994)
This report was a review of 1000+ patients suffering from various disorders (uterine bleeding, menopausal problems, PMS, mastodynia, hyper/poly-menorrhea). Treatments lasted up to 12 months. This study culminated experience with 3000+ patients suffering from PMS or CLI. Average treatment lasted 5 months.	"We believe that this short report, written by and intended for doctors in general and consulting practice, is well founded and will be of value. While we are deeply impressed by the dramatic advances of modern drug research, we cannot overlook the shadows of iatrogenic disease which lurk behind its successes. Practitioners naturally adopt a somewhat skeptical attitude towards highly potent drugs which have only recently come into use. We think it is appropriate to draw attention to this ancient and entirely harmless remedy."	Drs. Attelmann, Bends, Hellenkemper, and Warkall (1972)

(Table 9 continued on page 53)

TABLE 9, CONTINUED

Clinical Study Overview	Comments on Synthetic Hormone vs. Vitex Treatment	Physicians
This strict, long-term study recruited 15 women suffering from secondary amenorrhea due to CLI. Study lasted 6.5 months.	"Modern hormone treatment in gynecology has caused many well-proven remedies to be consigned to oblivion. The use of female sex hormones, however, is not without risk especially if continued for prolonged periods. As a result, there has been some obvious rethinking by physicians as well as patients. . . . even experts are now generally cautioning against an all too indiscriminate use of highly potent hormone preparations. The latter are likely to be indispensable in severe disorders. In milder, cases, however, Agnolyt (vitex) may, according to the present state of the art, be regarded as the treatment of choice."	Drs. Feldmann, Lamertz, and Bohnert (1990)
This long-term clinical study recruited 632 practicing gynecologists in the treatment of 2447 patients suffering from various cyclic disorders. Average treatment 6 months.	". . . Agnolyt (vitex) is highly recommended in the treatment of secondary amenorrhea . . . this is particularly true in comparison to the administering of gestagen, which provokes withdrawal bleedings, but does not lead to any change in the endogenous hormone production. Often, treatment with synthetic hormones only initiates bleeding and postpones finding the cause for the disorder." ". . . it is earnestly recommended that menstrual cyclic disorders are first treated with Agnolyt (vitex). This preparation offers high effectiveness, is greatly tolerated, is safe for long-term application, enhances the compliance of the patients, and is price competitive."	Drs. Lock and Kaiser (1990)

$\mathcal{R}$ECOMMENDED $\mathcal{R}$EADING

CONSTITUTIONAL TYPES AND TRADITIONAL CHINESE MEDICINE

Dharmananda, S. 1986. *Your Nature, Your Health*. Portland: Institute for Traditional Medicine and Preventive Health Care.

Hobbs, C. 1994. *Handbook for Herbal Healing*. Santa Cruz, CA: Botanica Press.

Kaptchuk, T.J. 1983. *The Web That Has No Weaver*. New York: Congdon & Weed, Inc.

Ladd, V. & D. Frawley. 1986. *The Yoga of Herbs*. Santa Fe: Lotus Press.

GENERAL WOMEN'S HEALTH

Gladstar, Rosemary. 1993. *Herbal Healing for Women*. New York: Simon & Schuster.

Scott, Julian & Susan. 1991. *Natural Medicine for Women*. New York, NY: Gaia Books.

Soule, Deb. 1995. *The Roots of Healing*. New York: Citadel Press.

Weed, Susun. 1996. *Breast Cancer? Breast Health! The Wise Woman Way*. Woodstock, NY: Ash Tree Publishing.

Hobbs, Christopher and Kathi Keville. Coming Fall 1996! Complete women's health and hormone book.

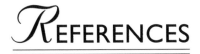

REFERENCES

Ainslie, W. 1826. *Materia Indica.* Reprinted by Neeraj Publishing House, Delhi.

Albus, G.A. 1966. Recurrent knee-joint discharge as a fragmental phenomenon of PMS. *Med. Welt.* 36: 1921-23.

Alleyne, J. 1733. *A New English Dispensatory.* London: Thomas Astley and S. Austen.

Amberg, D. R. 1994. Therapy of cyclical disorders with Vitex agnus-castus. *Zeitschrift fur Phytotherapy.* 15: 157-63.

Amman, V. 1975. Acne vulgaris and Agnus Castus. *Z. Allgemeinmed.* 51: 1645-48.

Amann, W. 1965. Beseitigung einer Obstipation with Agnolyt. *Therapy Gegenwart* 104: 1263-65.

Amann, W. 1967. A Look in the Abdominal Cavity. *Selecta* 16: 2982.

Amman, W. 1981. Post-Gestatory Acne. *Z. Allgemeinmed* 53: 295-98.

Amman, W. 1982. Amenorrea. *Z. Allgemeinmed* 58: 228-31.

Amman, W. & H. Kerres. 1964 Besserung der Stilleistung nach Gabe von Agnus castus. *Med. heute* 15: 1223.

Attelmann, H. & K. Bends. 1972. Agnolyt in the treatment of gynaecological complaints. *Zeitschrift Geriatrie.* 2: 239.

Attelmann, H., et al., 1972. Results of treatment of female disorders with Agnolyt. *Z. Praklin. Geriatr.* 2: 239-43.

Bautze, H. J. 1953. *Die Medizinische Welt* 5: 289.

Bensky, D. & A. Gamble. 1986. *Chinese Herbal Medicine Materia Medica.* Seattle: Eastland Press.

Bergner, P. 1990. Herbal Energetics. *Medical Herbalism* 2: 1: 6-7.

Berkow, R. 1992. *The Merck Manual of Diagnosis and Therapy.* 16th Edition. 1982. Merck & Co. 1662, 1685.

Binkley, S. A. 1995. *Endocrinology.* New York: HarperCollins.

Bleier, W. 1959. Phytotherapy in irregular menstrual cycles or bleeding periods and other gynecological disorders of endocrine origin. *Zentralblatt. Gynakol.* 81: 701-09.

Bonhert, K.G. et al. Phytotherapy in gynecology and obstetrics: *Vitex agnus castus. Erfahrungsheilkunde* 39: 494-502.

Brantner, F. 1979. Sexual hormones from plants in female medicine. *Ehk.* 28: 413.

Buchbauer, G. 1974. Iridoid und ihre pharmazeutische Bedeutung. O AZ 28. *Jg. Folge.* 10: 173-78.

Cahill, DJ., et al. 1994. Multiple follicular development associated with herbal medicine. *Human Reproduction.* 9: 1469-70.

Cazin, F.-J. 1886. *Plantes Médicinales.* Paris: Asselin & Houzeau.

Chadha, Y.R., chief ed. 1952-88. *The Wealth of India* (Raw Materials), 11 vols. New Delhi: Publications and Information Directorate, CSIR.

Coeugniet, E. et al. 1986. PMS and its Treatment. *Arztezeitchr Naturheilverf* 27: 619-22.

D. Roeder, Amberg. 1994. Treatment of Cyclical Disorders with Vitex agnus-castus. *Phytotherapie.* 157-63.

De Capite, L. 1967. Histology, anatomy, and antibiotic properties of Vitex agnus-castus. *Ann. Fac. Agr.* Univ. Studi Perugia 22: 109-26.

Dharmananda, S. 1986. *Your Nature, Your Health.* Portland: Institute for Traditional Medicine and Preventative Health Care.

Dittmar, F. W. 1989. Phytotherapie in der gynakologischen Praxis. *JiatrosGyna.* 5: 4-7.

Dittmar, F. W. 1992. Premenstrual syndrome: Treatment with a phytopharmaceutical. *TW Gynakol* 5: 60-68.

Du Mee, C. 1993. Vitex agnus castus. *Aust J Med Herbalism* 5: 63-65.

Duncan, A. 1788. *The Edinburgh New Dispensatory.* Edinburgh: William Creech.

Ecker, G. 1964. PMS als Schrittmacher einer pasttaumatischen Epilepsie. *Landarzt.* 40: 872-74. *Fac. Agr. Univ. Studi Perugia.* 22: 109-26.

Feldmann, H. U. et al. 1995. Therpaie der Gelbkorperschwache und des pramenstruellen Syndroms. Publication in process.

Felter, H.W. & J.U. Lloyd. 1898. *King's American Dispensatory.* Cincinatti: The Ohio Valley Co.

Foster, S. 1994. Chaste Tree Vitex Agnus-Castus. *Health Foods Business.* August: 26.

Gerard, J. 1633. *The Herbal or General History of Plants.* Reprinted by Dover Publications, New York (1975).

Giss, G. et al. 1968. Phytotherapeutische Behandlung der Akne. Z. Hautkr. *Geschlkrkh.* 43: 645-47.

Goebel, R. 1983. Vortage anlablich der III. wissenchaftl Tagung der Deutschen Gesellschart fur Senologie, Fulda.

Goerler, K. et al. 1985. Iridoid derivatives from Vitex agnus-castus. *Planta Med.* 6: 530-31.

Green, T. 1823. *The Universal Herbal.* London, Caxton Press.

Gregl, A. 1979. Die med. *Welt* 30: 264.

Gregl, A. 1982. Die med. *Welt* 33: 1641.

Grieve, M. (1976). 1931. *A Modern Herbal*. Middlesex, England: Penguin Books.

Hahn, G. et al. 1984. "Monk's Pepper." *Notabene medici*. 16: 233-36.

Halder, R. 1957. The Efficacy of Vitex Agnus Castus in womens health, specifically in the consideration of menstrual bleeding disorders. Inagural-Dissertation Tubingen.

Haller, J. 1959. Testierung von Gestagenen. *Therapiewoche*. 9: 481-84.

Hobbs, C.R. 1996. Author's observation.

Hooper, D. 1929. On Chinese medicine: drugs of Chinese pharmacies in Malaya. *The Gardens' Bulletin*, Straits Settlements (Singapore) 6: 1-165.

Hsu, H.-Y. 1986. *Oriental Materia Medica*. Long Beach: Oriental Healing Arts Institute.

Hyde, A.C. [d.m.]. Investigation of Vitex agnus castus. *The Herbal Practitioner* [v.m.]: 9-15.

James, R. 1747. *Pharmacopoeia Universalis: or a New Universal English Dispensatory*. London: for John Hodges, at the Looking-Glass.

Jones, W.H.S. 1956. Pliny: *Natural History*. Cambridge: Harvard University Press.

Kaptchuk, T.J. 1983. *The Web That Has No Weaver*. New York: Congdon & Weed, Inc.

Kayser, H.W. & S. Istanbulluoglu. 1954. Treatment of PMS without hormones. *Hippokrates* 25: 717.

Kelsey, H.P. & W.A. Dayton. 1942. *Standardized Plant Names*, 2nd ed. Harrisburg, PA: J. Horace McFarland Co.

Kleinman. et al. 1975. *Medicine in Chinese Cultures*. Washington: U.S. Department of Health, Education, and Welfare; National Institutes of Health.

Koch, F. E. 1954. Besizt Agnolyt eine Progestrone Wirkung Madaus Jahresbericht 8: 30.

Koch, H. [d.m.]. Vitex Agnus Castus L., unter Mitarbeit von Ulrike Vokovits.

Kubista, E. et al. 1986. *Gynakologische Rundschau* 26: 65.

Kustrak, K. et al. 1992. The composition of the essential oil of Vitex agnus castus. *Planta Medica*. 58 (suppl 1): A681.

Ladd, V. & D. Frawley. 1986. *The Yoga of Herbs*. Santa Fe: Lotus Press.

Larkey, S.V. & T. Pyles. 1941. *An Herbal* [1525]. New York: Scholars' Facsimiles & Reprints.

Lechmacher, A. 1968. Amdere Gynakologie. *Physik Med. Rehab*. 9: 211-14.

Levy, M. & N. Al-Khaledy. 1967. *The Medical Formulary of Al-Samarqandi*. Philadelphia: University of Pennsylvania Press.

Levy, M. 1966. *The Medical Formulary or Aqrabadhin of Al-Kindi.* Madison: University of Wisconsin Press.

Lifschutz, A. 1941. Prevention of experimental uterine and extrauterine fibroids by testosterone and progestone. *Endorcrin.* 28: 669-75.

Lindner, F. 1972. Illnesses of the vegetative nervous system. *Naturheilpraxis* 25: 460.

List, P.H. & L. Hörhammer. 1973. *Hagers Handbuch der Pharmazeutischen Praxis,* 7 vols. New York: Springer-Verlag.

Loch, E. G. et al. 1989. Dyshormal Menstrual Bleeding Disorders: Diagnosis and Therapy. *Gynakologie.* 2: 379-85.

Loch, E. G. et al. 1990. Diagnosis and Treatment of Dyshormonal Bleeding. *Gynakol Prax.* 14: 489-95.

Loch, E. G. et al. 1991. Treatment of Menstrual Disturbances with Vitex agnus castus tincture. 1991. *Der Frauenartz.* 32: 867-70.

Loch, E. G. 1990. Diagnosis and Treatment of Dyshormonal Menstrual Periods in the General Practice. *Arztezeitschr. Naturheilverf.* 31: 455-58.

Madaus, G. 1938. *Handbook of Biological Medicine.* Reprinted by Georg Olms Verlag, NY (1976).

Madaus & Co. 1994. Medicine from Nature. 'Agnolyt' the natural way for hormone balance. Cologne: Dr. Madaus & Co.

Milewicz, A. et al. 1993. Vitex agnus castus extracts in the treatment of luteal phase defects due to hyperprolactinemia: Results of a randomized placebo-controlled double-blind study. *Arzneim-Forsch Drug Res* 43: 752-56.

Mishurova, S.S. et al. 1986. Essential oil of Vitex agnus castus L., its fractional composition and antimicrobial activity. *Rastit. Resur.* 22: 526-30.

Mohr, H. 1954. Clinical study on the promotion of lactation. *Dtsch. Med. Wschr.* 41: 1513-16.

Ortiz de Urbina, A.V. et al. 1994. In vitro antispasmodic activity of peracetylated penstemonoside, acubin and catalpol. *Planta Medica,* 60: 512-15.

Perry, L.M. 1980. *Medicinal Plants of East and Southeast Asia.* Cambridge: The MIT Press.

Peters-Welte, C. & M. Albrecht. 1994. Menstrual Abnormalities and PMS. *TW Gynakologie.* 7: 49-52.

Polunin, O. 1987. *Flowers of Greece and the Balkans.* New York: Oxford University Press.

Porppings, D. et al. 1988. Diagnostic and therapy of corpus luteum deficiency in practice. *Therapiewoche* 38: 2992-3001.

Probst, V. & O.A. Roth. 1954. [t.m.] *Dtsch. Med. Wschr.* 35: 1271-74.

Proppings, D. et al. 1987. Treatment of corpus luteum deficiency. *Z. Allgemeinmed.* 63: 932-33.

Proppings, D. et al. 1988. Diagnostic and therapy of corpus luteum deficiency in practice. *Therapiewoche* 38: 2992-3001.

Razzack, H.M.A. 1980. The concept of birth control in Unani medical literature. Unpublished manuscript of the author, 64 pp.

Recio, MC. et al. 1994. Structural considerations on the iridoids as anti-inflammatory agents. *Planta Medica.* 60: 232-34.

Rehder, A. 1927. *Manual of Cultivated Trees and Shrubs.* New York: Macmillan & Co.

Revolutionary Health Committee of Hunan Province. 1977. *A Barefoot Doctor's Manual.* Seattle: Madrona Publishers.

Roth, O. A. 1956. *Med. Klinik.* 51: 1263.

Sliutz, G. et al. 1993. Agnus castus extracts inhibit prolactin secretion of rat pituitary cells. *Hormone and Metabolic Research.* 25: 253-55.

Smith, F.P. & G.A. Stuart, translators and annotators. 1976. *Chinese Medicinal Herbs* (derived from the *Pen T'sao* of Li Shih-chen, 1578). San Francisco: Georgetown Press.

Steinegger, E. & R. Hansel. 1988. *Handbook of Pharmacognosy and Phytopharmacy.* New York: Springer-Verlag.

Suh, NJ, et al. 1991. Pharmacokinetic study of an iridoid glucoside: aucubin. *Pharmaceutical Research,* 8: 1059-63.

Tierra, M. 1988. *Planetary Herbology.* Santa Fe: Lotus Press.

Urdang, G. 1944. *Pharmacopoeia Londinensis of 1618* reproduced in facsimile. Madison: State Historical Society of Wisconsin.

Utian, WH. 1990. *Managing Your Menopause.* Englewood Cliffs, NJ: Simon and Schuster Fireside Press.

Wollenweber, E. & K. Mann. 1983. Flavonols from fruits of Vitex agnus castus. *Planta Med.* 48: 126-27.

Wood, H.C. & J.P. Remington. 1894. *The Dispensatory of the United States of America,* 17th ed. Philadelphia: J.B. Lippincoat Co.

Wuttke, W. 1992. Zellbiologische Untersuchungen mit Agnolyt-Preparationen (NIH 246, NIH 247). Personl. Mitteilung.

Yamazaki, M., et al. 1994. Promotion of neuronal differentiation of PC12h cells by natural lignans and iridoids. *Biological and Pharmaceutical Bulletin.* 17: 1604-8.